Helping Children with Life-Threatening Medical Issues

CHARITY & PHILANTHROPY
UNLEASHED

Joanne
Mattern

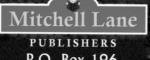

Mitchell Lane
PUBLISHERS
P.O. Box 196
Hockessin, DE 19707

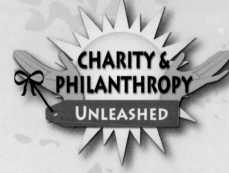

Mitchell Lane

PUBLISHERS

CHARITY & PHILANTHROPY

UNLEASHED

Conquering Disease

Emergency Aid

Environmental Protection

Helping Children with Life-Threatening Medical Issues

Helping Our Veterans

Preserving Human Rights Around the World

The Quest to End World Hunger

Support for Education

PUBLISHER'S NOTE: The facts in this book have been thoroughly researched. Documentation of such research can be found on pages 44–45. While every possible effort has been made to ensure accuracy, the publisher will not assume liability for damages caused by inaccuracies in the data, and makes no warranty on the accuracy of the information contained herein.

The Internet sites referenced herein were active as of the publication date. Due to the fleeting nature of some web sites, we cannot guarantee that they will all be active when you are reading this book.

Printing 1   2   3   4   5   6   7   8   9

Library of Congress
Cataloging-in-Publication Data

Mattern, Joanne, 1963–
  Helping children with life-threatening medical issues / by Joanne Mattern.
       pages cm. — (Charity and philanthropy unleashed)
  Includes glossary.
  Includes bibliographical references and index.
  Audience: 9-13
  Grades: 4-8
  ISBN 978-1-61228-571-9 (library bound)
  1. Sick children—Services for. I. Title.
  HV687.M38 2015
  362.19892—dc23
                                              2014008298

eBook ISBN: 9781612286099

PBP

·Contents

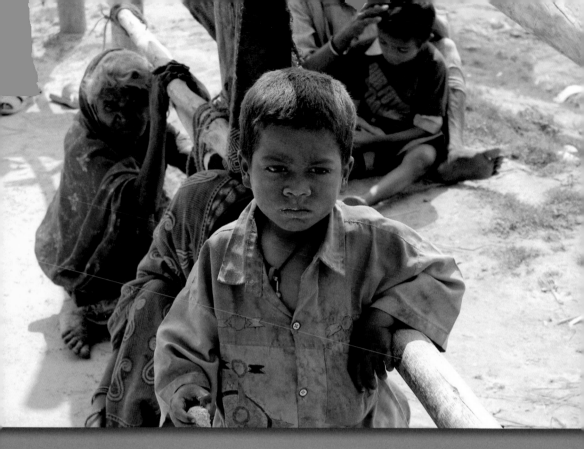

Introduction

Illness, injury, and death are sad facts of life everywhere on Planet Earth. While most of us are lucky enough to enjoy good health and a happy life, millions more children suffer every day.

Millions of children are born in countries filled with poverty and warfare. These conditions prevent children from receiving good nutrition or necessary medicines. A doctor might be miles away, if a doctor can be found at all. For children in these countries, even a minor illness can turn into something deadly. Children who live in poverty or war zones get sick more easily. They can also contract diseases that are very rare in the United States. Without the medicine to help them, children die every day.

It isn't only children in faraway lands who suffer. Children all over the United States and Canada have problems too. Even though the United States and Canada are highly developed countries with many programs to help sick children and their families, many children still suffer from illnesses and chronic conditions, such as asthma, which is a respiratory disease that makes it hard to breathe. Even tooth decay can be a huge problem in areas where it isn't so easy to go to the dentist. Children live in poverty even in your community. It's a sad fact that not every child has access to good health care or dental care.

It isn't only poor children who have medical problems. A serious illness, injury, or birth defect can strike any family at any time. For these children, medical help is needed right away. But how can families find the help they need?

Fortunately for children and families all over the world, there are many organizations whose sole purpose is to help sick families. Some of these organizations make life better for sick children by granting wishes and creating once-in-a-lifetime experiences. Other organizations visit children in hospitals or create a home away from home where a family can relax and experience normal life while still being close to a hospitalized child.

Hospitals help too. Many hospitals have created cutting-edge medical programs to help ill or injured children. At some of these hospitals, children receive the best medical care free of charge—all because caring people decided to help.

Other organizations take a broader approach. Global organizations such as UNICEF and Save the Children strive to improve conditions all over the world by wiping out illnesses and providing medical care for children who would otherwise have no way to see a doctor.

In this book, you'll discover some of the organizations and people who are working tirelessly to make the world a better place for children with medical needs. You'll also find out how you can help in ways both big and small. Sometimes the best medicine is just someone reaching out a helping hand.

CHAPTER 1

Batkid Makes a Wish

Early in the morning of November 15, 2013, an urgent message went out to residents of the San Francisco area. The city's police chief asked if anyone knew where Batkid was because the city needed his help to solve some serious crimes. Soon afterward, Batkid—the secret identity of a five-year-old boy named Miles Scott—was in the city and ready for action.

Batkid teamed up with Batman and climbed into the superhero's car, the Batmobile. Quickly they raced to the Hyde Street cable car line where they found a damsel in distress tied up on the tracks. Batkid helped Batman untie the woman before the cable car came along. Hundreds of people watched from the sidewalks and cheered the little superhero as he saved the day.

But Batkid's work wasn't done yet. Another message came in from police, announcing that one of Batman's archenemies, the Riddler, was robbing a bank. Once again, Batkid and Batman rushed to the scene of the crime where they caught the Riddler red-handed and saved the day in front of another cheering crowd.

Then it was time for a break. Batkid and Batman stopped at a local restaurant for some hamburgers and superhero conversation. But another crime was in the works. Just as they finished lunch, an urgent message came in from the chief of police telling Batkid to look out the window. There he saw a huge crowd of people jumping up and down and yelling for help. It turned out that the Penguin, another classic villain, was kidnapping Lou Seal, the famous mascot of the city's baseball team, the San Francisco Giants. Once again, Batkid and Batman jumped into the Batmobile

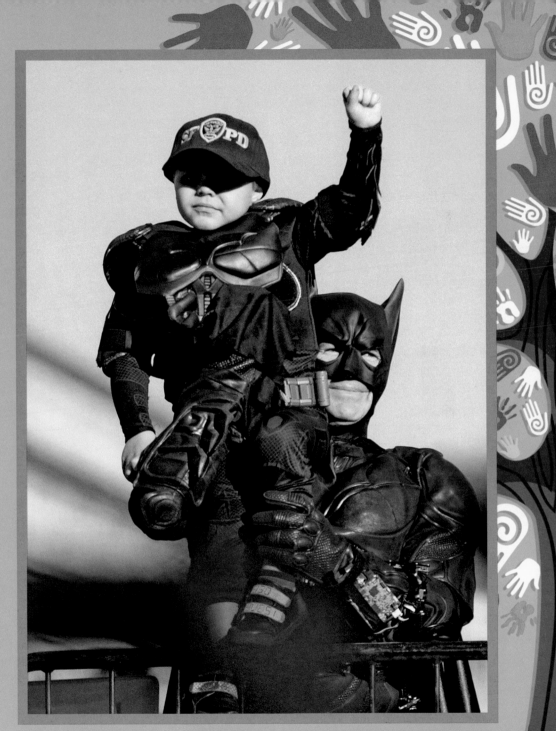

Batman holds up Batkid Miles Scott in front of a cheering crowd in San Francisco after the two saved the city as part of a Make-a-Wish event on November 15, 2013. Miles, who lives in Tulelake, California, has battled leukemia since he was a toddler and had his biggest wish—to be Batkid— come true.

The major of San Francisco presents Miles "Batkid" Scott with the key to the city after the little superhero saved the day as part of a Make-a-Wish event.

and sped off to the ballpark. Thanks to their quick work, the Penguin was captured and Lou Seal was saved.

With the city's crime wave stopped in its tracks, it was time to celebrate. Batkid went to City Hall where San Francisco's mayor and police chief thanked the little boy for his hard work. They also presented Batkid and his younger brother with special keys to the city—keys made of chocolate! The *San Francisco Chronicle* printed a special newspaper that day describing all of Batkid's heroic achievements. The headline read, "Batkid Saves City."[1] Batkid also received thousands of messages on Twitter and other social media sites. Even President Barack Obama got involved, posting a short video on Twitter to say, "Way to go, Batkid. Way to save Gotham City."

Why did San Francisco go to so much trouble to transform itself into Gotham City and set up crimes for Batkid to solve? It was all to make a sick child have the best day of his life. Miles Scott—the real Batkid—is a five-year-old boy who has battled a form of cancer called leukemia since he was eighteen months old. An organization called the Make-a-Wish Foundation asked Miles what he would like most in the world. Miles' answer was to be Batkid for a day. "He is a sunny, positive little boy and finds his inspiration in superheroes," the Foundation said about Miles. "When we interviewed Miles for a wish, he surprised even his parents: He wishes to be Batkid!"[2]

As it does with thousands of other wishes every year, the Make-a-Wish Foundation set about granting Miles' wish. San Francisco, which had worked with Make-a-Wish before, was happy to help.

"This is one that we thought of as a great opportunity for people to share in the power of a wish so they can see how it affects not only the children and their families, but also the other people involved," Jen Wilson, the marketing and promotions manager for Make-a-Wish in San Francisco, told ABCNews.com. "It has a big impact on many people. Since he wants to be a superhero, we felt like having a large crowd there waiting with

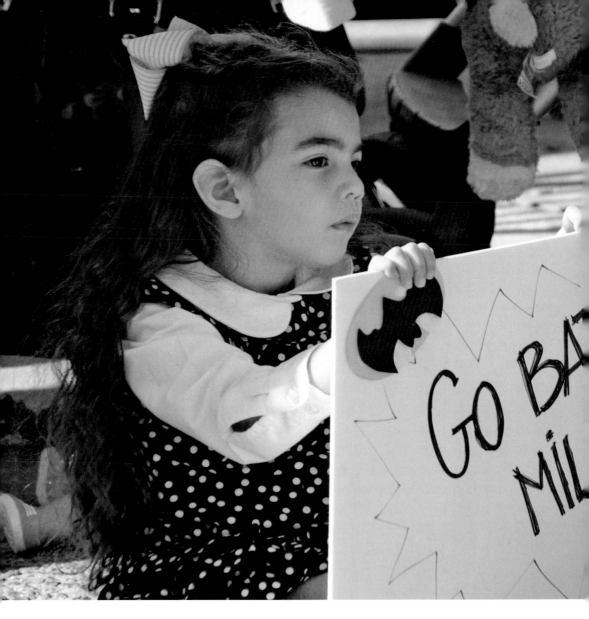

signs and cheering him on would make him feel like a hero, not just because he battles villains and helped fight crime, but he's a true hero."[3] So Make-a-Wish asked for volunteers to play the parts of Batman, the Riddler, the Penguin, and other characters, as well as the crowd that cheers Batkid on. They expected about a hundred people to volunteer. Then something unusual happened. Miles' story went viral. Suddenly Twitter was blazing with the hashtag #SFBatKid. Facebook and other social media sites reported on the story. Soon thousands of people were volunteering to help.

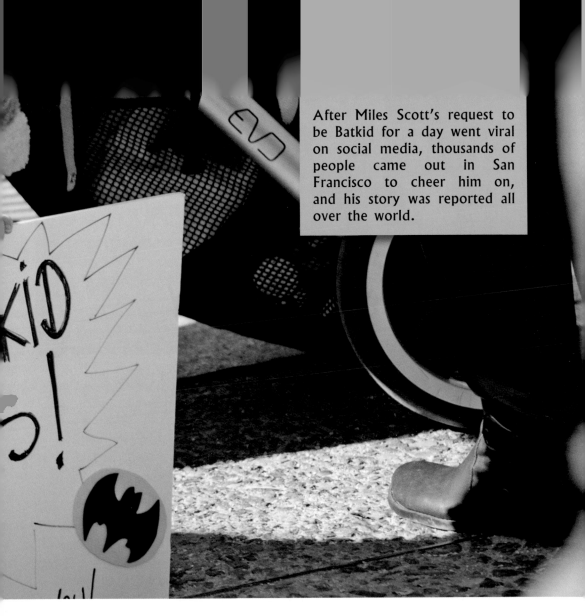

After Miles Scott's request to be Batkid for a day went viral on social media, thousands of people came out in San Francisco to cheer him on, and his story was reported all over the world.

Batkid's experience was unusual for Make-a-Wish. As Jen Wilson admitted, "This is definitely not the typical wish we grant."[4] Still, Batkid's adventures had an important result. Helping Miles and viewing his story made a lot of people feel good. These people discovered that helping sick children is an important and wonderful thing to do. Also many people found out about the work of the Make-a-Wish Foundation, which has dedicated itself to granting wishes to sick children for many years.

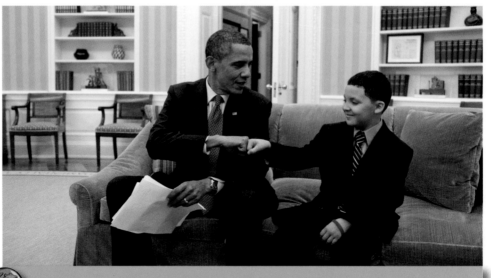

The Make-a-Wish Foundation made Diego Diaz's wish come true. The boy got to meet—and fist-bump! —President Barack Obama during a visit to the Oval Office on June 23, 2011.

The Make-a-Wish Foundation got a lot of publicity on November 15, 2013, but it has been helping children in ways big and small for more than thirty years. Make-a-Wish is not the only organization that helps sick children. There are many other places, organizations, and people who work tirelessly so sick children can have the best care and the best chance at life. There are hospitals where desperately ill children can receive the best medical care for free. Foundations raise awareness of different diseases while providing support to families and funds to doctors to research new treatments. International organizations work to wipe out diseases all over the world, while many large corporations donate money and encourage their employees to donate their time to make life better for children in need.

There are so many children and families who need help and so many people who are willing to provide that help. In this book, you'll learn more about these organizations and how they are changing the world, one child at a time. You'll also learn what you can do to help.

Who Pays for Wishes?

Filling Miles Scott's Batkid wish was not cheap. The city of San Francisco spent $105,000 on November 15, mostly to set up video and other communications equipment and for crowd control. The city was prepared to pay the bill, until a generous couple who run a foundation stepped forward and paid it instead.[5]

   Most Make-a-Wish projects aren't nearly as big or expensive as Miles' was. Many children wish to meet celebrities or be police officers or firefighters for a day. The people who help make these wishes come true donate their time and don't expect to get paid. Other wishes involve trips, which are paid for by Make-a-Wish itself. The foundation is supported by donations from the public and from corporations, along with fundraising events such as parties and dinners. The Make-a-Wish Foundation estimates that the average cost of fulfilling a wish is $7500.[6]

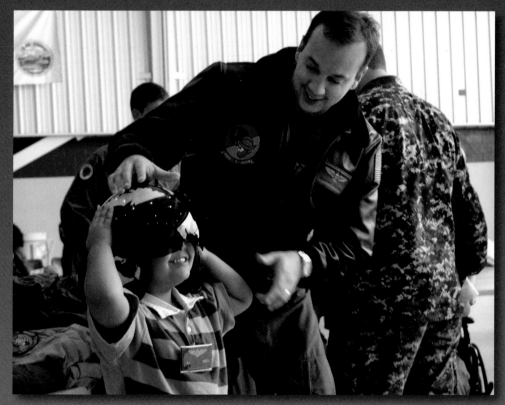

The Make-a-Wish Foundation has been granting wishes since 1981 and thousands of people have helped make children's wishes come true. Here, children enjoy an exciting visit to the Logistics Support Squadron in California, where they receive an inside look at life in the military.

CHAPTER 2

Saving Young Lives Around the World

Every day, thousands of children around the world die of preventable causes. Some die of hunger. Others die of diseases for which there are treatments and cures. The problem is that many children in other countries, and even in the United States, do not have access to good medical care.

For centuries, people have been working to make medical care available to the most poverty-stricken places. These organizations bring medicine and staff, and they work to educate people about how to prevent illness and make sick children well again.

The World Health Organization

The United Nations is an international organization that works to improve living conditions for people around the world. Since this is a big job, the United Nations has many different divisions. The World Health Organization is part of the United Nations.

The World Health Organization, or WHO, was formed in 1948. Its original goals were to control the spread of malaria and tuberculosis, to improve the health of mothers and children around the world, and to improve nutrition and environmental hygiene.[1]

Over the past fifty-five years, WHO has helped eradicate a disease called smallpox. When WHO started its efforts against smallpox in 1958, more than two million people died of this disease every year.[2] The last natural case of smallpox was reported in 1977, making it the first disease to be eliminated by human efforts.[3] WHO has also worked to prevent polio, measles, AIDS,

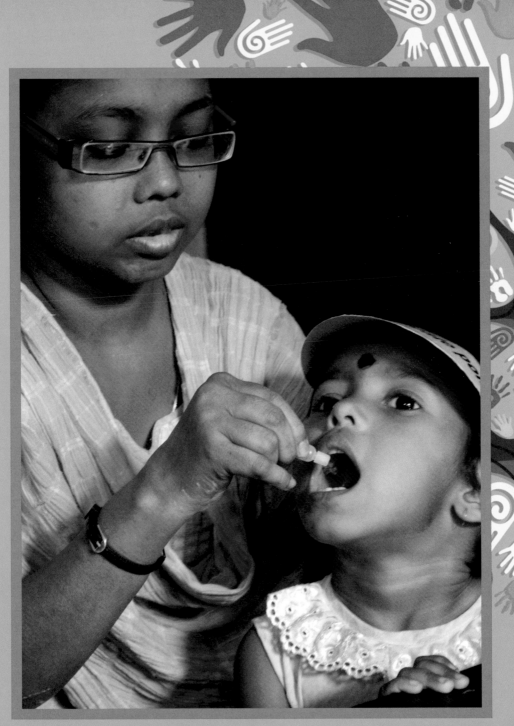

A child is vaccinated against polio during a campaign in Kolkata, India. Although most polio cases only occur in just ten countries, the disease can easily spread across national borders. That's why it is important to vaccinate children all over the world to prevent the spread of disease.

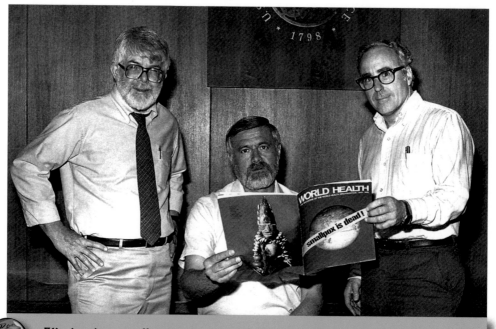

Eliminating smallpox was one of the greatest medical achievements in the 20th century. This 1980 photograph shows three former directors of the Global Smallpox Eradication Program as they read the news that smallpox has been officially wiped out.

tuberculosis, and malaria through vaccination and public health education, as well as calling for better nutrition and environmental conditions for people around the world. These efforts have created better health for children—and adults—all over the globe.

The World Health Organization is not the only part of the United Nations focused on children. UNICEF, or the United Nations International Children's Emergency Fund, began in 1946 to help children in Europe after World War II. Over the years, UNICEF has expanded to 190 countries where it helps children's medical needs as well as fighting against malnutrition, lack of health education, poverty, and disaster relief.[4]

Save the Children International

Save the Children calls itself "the world's leading independent organization for children."[5] Its goal is to save children's lives,

SAVING YOUNG LIVES AROUND THE WORLD

fight for their rights, and make sure each child realizes his or her full potential. Save the Children works in 120 countries around the world.[6]

One of Save the Children's main goals is improving children's health. The organization states that seven million children around the world die before their fifth birthday.[7] To change this, Save the Children provides medical care to children and trains local residents to be health-care providers and educators.

Save the Children is working with governments as the focus of its Every One campaign because it believes that achieving its goals is impossible without government cooperation. The organization states, "These deaths are not random events beyond our control . . . they are the outcome of policy and political choices taken by governments"[8] as well as cultural beliefs. Save the Children aims to address the underlying causes of newborn and child mortality, which it lists as poverty, discrimination, conflict, the denial of rights, and barriers to equal access to health care. In doing so, Save the Children hopes to make life better for children all over the world.

The Measles and Rubella Initiative

You probably have bad memories of getting vaccinations at the doctor's office. Having a needle stuck into your arm is not much fun, especially for babies and young children. However, vaccinations have saved the lives of millions of people by preventing diseases that once claimed many lives.

If you read a medical book from sixty or seventy years ago, you'll find descriptions of diseases you've probably never heard of today. Measles, polio, scarlet fever, rheumatic fever, diphtheria—all these diseases were once very common and extremely deadly. During the 1950s and earlier, it was not uncommon for children to die of these diseases or endure weeks of illness and pain. Some children who survived were left with lifelong disabilities, such as paralyzed limbs, deafness, or serious heart conditions.

Chapter 2

Over the past seventy years, children in the United States have received a number of different vaccinations to prevent diseases that were once very common. It's pretty clear that vaccinations have improved public health and saved many lives.

Things are very different in other parts of the world, however. Measles is one example of a disease that has almost disappeared in the United States and other Western nations but is still a problem in other parts of the world. According to the Measles and Rubella Initiative, measles is one of the most contagious diseases ever known.[9] Measles is caused by a virus and spreads through coughing and sneezing. Up to 90 percent of the people who come in contact with someone who has measles will catch the disease.[10] The symptoms of the measles are a high fever, a rash, and a bad cough. Because the measles also weakens the body's immune system, about 30 percent of people with the measles can also get very sick from complications, such as pneumonia or diarrhea.[11] Before the year 2000, more than 535,000 children worldwide died from measles or measles complications every year.[12]

Another form of measles is rubella, which is also known as German measles. Rubella is usually a minor illness, but if a woman catches rubella while she is pregnant, she has a high risk of giving birth to a child with serious birth defects such as blindness, deafness, or heart problems. More than 100,000 children are born with complications from rubella every year.[13]

In 2000, the Measles and Rubella Initiative began when a number of American and international aid organizations got together with the goal of eradicating measles around the world. The founding members of the Initiative included the American Red Cross, the United Nations Foundation, the US Centers for Disease Control and Prevention, UNICEF, and the World Health Organization. The Initiative came up with a simple combined vaccine that prevents both measles and rubella and costs just one dollar. The Initiative calls this vaccine "one of the most cost-effective health interventions available."[14]

Mongolian street children eat lunch at a Save the Children day shelter in Ulan Bataar, Mongolia in October 2000. Save the Children provides a place for these children to get a good meal, have a warm, safe place to stay, and receive medical care they otherwise would not be able to get because they are poor and homeless.

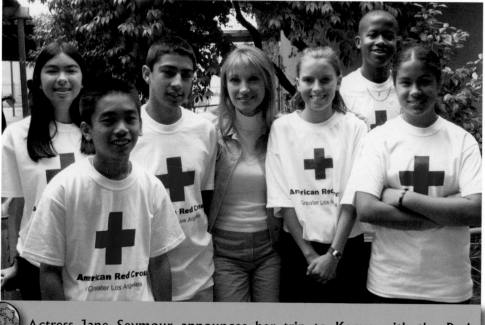

Actress Jane Seymour announces her trip to Kenya with the Red Cross and six US teenagers on a Measles Initiative vaccination campaign.

In the years since the Measles and Rubella Initiative began, more than 1.1 billion doses of the vaccine have been delivered to children in eighty countries. Today 84 percent of children are vaccinated against measles. As a result, deaths from the measles are down by more than 70 percent.[15]

The Measles and Rubella Initiative works with the governments of different countries in order to make the vaccine available. These partnerships have had amazing results. According to the Initiative, measles deaths in Africa have dropped by 84 percent in ten years, and deaths in Asian countries dropped by 82 percent between 2009 and 2012.[16] The countries in North, South, and Central America have almost eliminated measles and rubella completely, although some cases do occur if people have contact with others who have the measles. The goal is to completely eliminate measles by 2020. Doing so will prevent an estimated 13.4 million deaths, most of them children.[17]

If We Have Vaccines, Why Do People Still Get Sick?

If a person is immune to measles or another disease, he or she will not get the disease. There are two major ways to develop immunity. The most common is to be vaccinated against the disease. The other way is to have the disease. In both cases, the body creates antibodies to fight the disease, which means the person won't get sick if he or she is exposed to the disease again.

However, even though most people in the United States and Europe are vaccinated against measles and rubella, people do still get the disease. This happens when an unvaccinated person comes in contact with someone who has the measles. For example, a person in New York City might visit a foreign country and come into contact with someone who has the measles. If that New Yorker is not immune to the measles, he or she is likely to not only develop the disease but also spread it to any other unvaccinated person in the United States that he or she comes in contact with. Another way measles can spread is if a person with the measles travels to another country by airplane and infects many of the people he or she comes in contact with on the plane. These chances are why many doctors and governments insist that everyone get vaccinated against diseases.

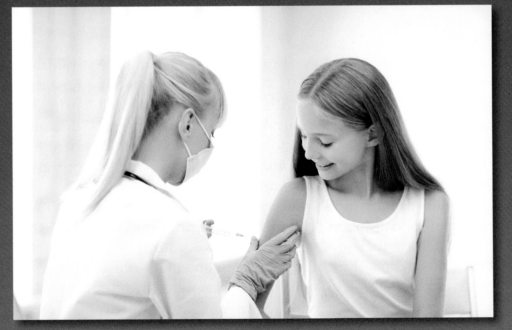

Young teen receiving vaccination.

CHAPTER 3

Medical Research and Care

If you're sick or in an accident, your parents will probably take you to the doctor or even to the local hospital. But what happens when children get really sick? What happens to families when children are struck with a serious illness such as cancer, or they are burned in a fire, badly injured in an accident, or born with birth defects that seem impossible to overcome? The good news is that there are hospitals that take special care of the youngest and most seriously ill patients—sometimes for free! In doing so, they help make life better not just for those children, but for their families and for other children who will face the same problems in the future.

St. Jude's

In February 1962, a new hospital named St. Jude Children's Research Hospital opened in Memphis, Tennessee. The hospital's goal was to treat children with "catastrophic illnesses," primarily cancer. At that time, the survival rate for children with cancer was extremely low. The doctors at St. Jude wanted to change all that. They did so in a way that would help patients both at St. Jude and at other hospitals around the world.

St. Jude is one of the most important centers for research and treatment of childhood cancers in the world. Children are referred to St. Jude by their doctors. If they have a form of cancer that is being researched at St. Jude's and are accepted into the program, these children receive some of the best care in the world. They are treated with new medicines and procedures that aren't available anywhere else.

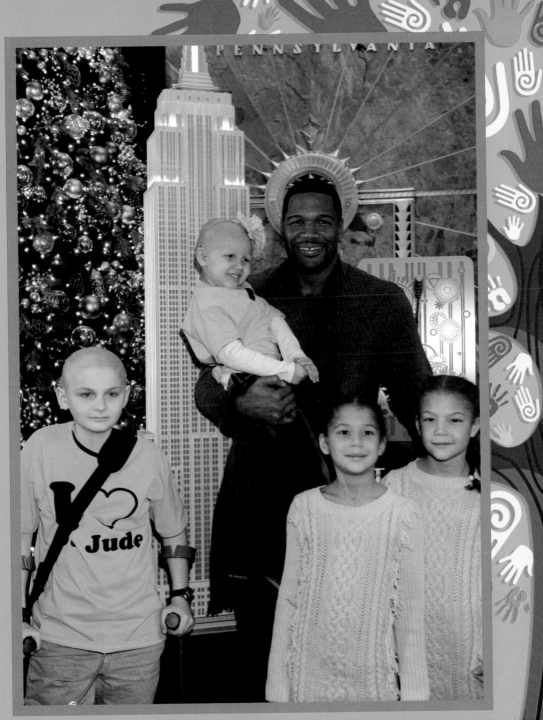

Many celebrities are happy to donate their time and talents to help sick children. Football star and talk-show host Michael Strahan and his daughters joined patients from St. Jude Children's Research Hospital to light New York City's Empire State Building green in celebration of the hospital's "Thanks and Giving" campaign in December 2012.

The doctors at St. Jude publish everything they learn in medical journals and spread the news of their work around the world. St. Jude makes their research available for free to anyone who wants to use it. This access to information has allowed doctors all over the world to use new cancer treatments that have saved many lives.

According to St. Jude's website, the survival rate for acute lymphoblastic leukemia—the most common form of childhood cancer—was only four percent in 1962. Today the survival rate is 94 percent. Overall survival rates for all childhood cancers have risen from 20 percent in 1962 to 80 percent today.[1]

One of the most amazing facts about St. Jude is that all of the patients who go there are treated absolutely free. Their families do not have to pay anything for their medical care. St. Jude has a daily operating cost of almost two million dollars, which is all raised through donations.[2] Through the generosity of St. Jude's founders, doctors, and supporters, this hospital has changed lives for millions of families.

Shriners Hospitals

The Shriners is an organization of men who get together for fun and fellowship. This organization also does a lot of fundraising for good causes. Their most famous contribution to helping sick children is the system of Shriners Hospitals in North America.

The first Shriners Hospital was founded in Shreveport, Louisiana, in 1922 and cared for orthopedic patients.[3] Today there are twenty-two Shriners Hospitals in the United States, Canada, and Mexico.[4] All these hospitals treat children for free. Families come from all over for treatment, and the Shriners even pay for their transportation. These hospitals have created research and treatment procedures that have led to improved care for children with specific medical conditions all over the world.

Over the years, Shriners hospitals have treated children with birth defects such as clubfoot, dwarfism, cerebral palsy, and other conditions that affect bones and muscles. Shriners Hospitals not

Children at Shriners Hospitals receive lots of support from the community. Here, two US Navy reservists visit a young patient at the Shriners Hospital in Portland, Oregon. The reservists and their ship were in town as part of the city's famous Rose Bowl Parade.

only offer treatment and therapy for children with orthopedic needs, they also have their own labs to create custom-made prosthetics, braces, and other equipment to help patients walk and use their limbs again.

In 1962, the Shriners established three hospitals to treat burn patients.[5] Burns are one of the most severe injuries a person can suffer, and recovering is a long and extremely painful process.

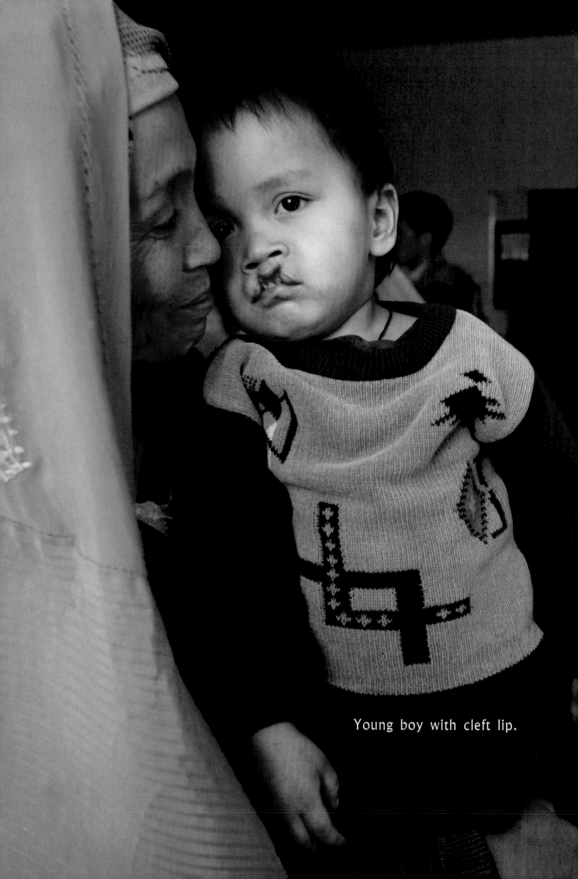

Young boy with cleft lip.

Today the main treatment for burns is grafting healthy skin to replace the skin that was destroyed by the burns. The doctors at Shriners made many advancements in skin grafts as well as the development of artificial skin. Shriners helps burn patients regain movement of damaged body parts through physical therapy and works on ways to reduce scars left by burn injuries.

Shriners Hospitals also treat spinal cord injuries, which affect a child's ability to walk, move, and even breathe. Shriners Hospitals developed the first spinal cord injury rehabilitation centers in the United States designed specifically for children that can help them regain movement and return home to live an active and healthy life.

The final medical need treated at Shriners is a birth defect known as cleft lip and palate. In this condition, the palate, or roof of a child's mouth, does not form completely. This results in a lip that is "split," as well as a palate that is open all the way into the sinuses. Cleft palate can cause serious problems with eating, speaking, tooth development, and hearing. At Shriners, young patients receive surgery, therapy, and dental work to help them have a normal appearance and function.

Olivia Stamps seemed like a normal child—until she learned to walk and her parents and doctor noticed she walked on her toes. Soon afterward, Olivia was diagnosed with a condition called cerebral palsy, which affects the body's muscles. She traveled to Shriners for treatment. Shriners used cutting-edge technology called movement analysis, using electronic sensors and high-speed cameras to create images of exactly how Olivia moved and then analyzing the data on computers to create the best treatment plan for her. Olivia said, "My dream was about trying to get my legs fixed so one day I could fit in with all the other kids and it came true. I can run, play, do whatever I want."[6]

Brendon Wisely lost his left leg in a lawn mower accident. Brendon was fitted with a prosthesis, or artificial limb, but the leg didn't fit right. Then Brendon and his family were referred to Shriners, where Brendon was given a prosthetic leg created just

A young orthopedic patient accompanies Navy Rear Admiral Bill Goodwin on a special tour of the Shriners Hospital for Children in Greenville, South Carolina, in October 2009. Goodwin's visit is an example of how the members of the military and other citizens help children with serious medical needs.

for him. Brendon became one of the top ten race drivers in his competition group, racing against drivers who did not have any disabilities. Brendon's father says that Shriners doesn't believe in a child with a disability. Brendon himself says, "Shriners are the only reason I am able to race. They save lives and make little children smile when no one else can. To me they are angels on Earth!"[7]

A Seven-Dollar Promise

St. Jude was started by an entertainer named Danny Thomas. About seventy years ago, Thomas was struggling to make a living as an entertainer and also support his wife, who was expecting a baby. Thomas was so worried about how he would pay the hospital bills for his daughter's birth that he visited a church and put his last seven dollars in the collection box as he prayed for a way to pay his bills. The next day, Thomas received an acting job that would cover his expenses. Two years later, Thomas was struggling again. Remembering his experience in the church, he prayed to St. Jude, who is considered the patron saint of hopeless causes by Catholics. Thomas made a simple promise: "Help me find my way in life and I will build you a shrine."[8]

Soon Thomas's career was going very well, and over the next few years he became one of America's most popular entertainers, even starring in his own television show. In the early 1950s, Thomas began planning and raising money for a shrine to St. Jude. In 1955, Thomas and some friends and business owners in Memphis decided to create a hospital that would treat children with cancer and other deadly diseases. Their goal was to create a research center for the children of the world. St. Jude Children's Research Hospital opened in 1962. Over the past fifty years, the hospital has improved health care and survival rates for children, all because a struggling actor kept a promise.

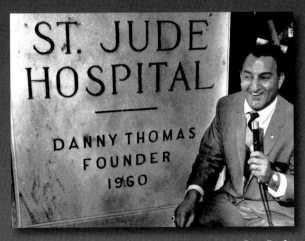

Entertainer Danny Thomas opens St. Jude Children's Research Hospital in Memphis, Tennessee, on February 4, 1962. Thomas and his friends raised several million dollars to start the hospital, which continues to help young cancer patients through generous donations.

CHAPTER 4

Fulfilling Wishes

Sometimes when you're sick, all you have are your dreams. You might be tired all the time, or be in pain or feel like throwing up. You might not be able to play with your friends, go to school, or take part in sports or hobbies. You might wish for something really wonderful to happen to you. Luckily for sick children around the world, there are many organizations that work hard to make those wonderful wishes and dreams come true, just like the Make a Wish Foundation made Miles Scott's wish to be Batkid come true.

The Starlight Foundation

Another well-known organization is the Starlight Foundation which began in 1982 by a filmmaker named Peter Samuelson and his cousin, actress Emma Samms. Emma had lost her younger brother to illness when they were children and had made a point of visiting sick children and doing what she could to brighten their day. One day, Emma visited a young boy named Sean who was seriously ill with a brain tumor. Sean dreamed of going to Disneyland, so Peter and Emma fulfilled his wish and brought him and his mom on a magical trip.[1]

Although Starlight began strictly as a wish-granting organization, it soon became something bigger. Starlight became known as a leader in creating family-centered programs for sick children. These programs help families with hospitalized children cope with the challenges of a medical journey in many different ways. Starbright World, a project of Starlight, is the first-ever social network for teens with chronic and life-threatening medical

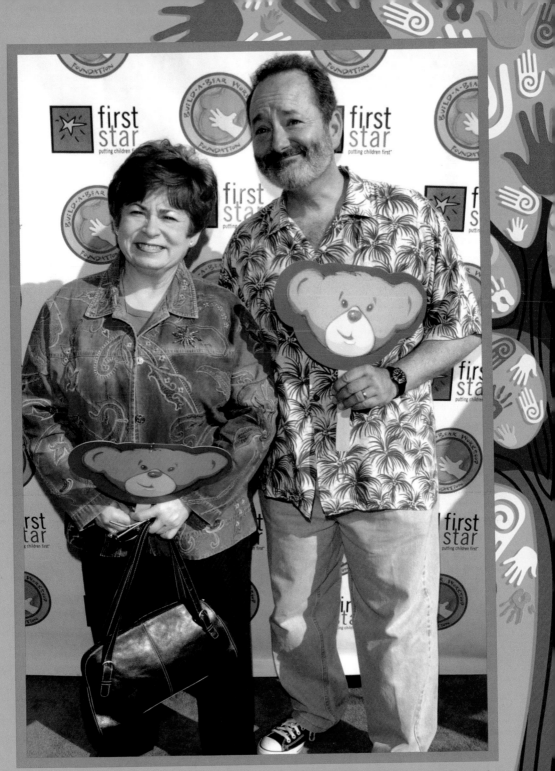

Maxine Clark and Peter Samuelson appear at a benefit for the Starlight Foundation in Santa Monica, California.

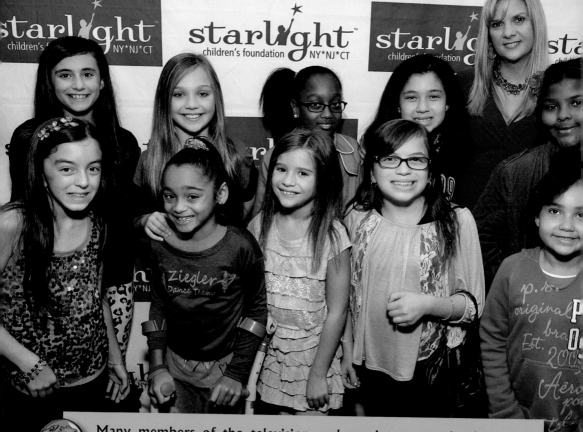

Many members of the television and movie community help the Starlight Foundation bring joy to sick children. Here, young dancers from the TV show Dance Moms pose with children from the Starlight Foundation at an event in New York City in September 2012.

conditions and their siblings. Starlight Fun Centers are mobile entertainment systems that are brought into hospitals to provide children with therapeutic play and fun. The PC Pals program provides laptop computers to young hospital patients, allowing them to play games, watch videos, and enjoy social media instead of focusing on their illness.[2]

Starlight also works with doctors and hospital staff to make the scary world of medicine more kid-friendly and understandable. The Starlight Tablet and Hospital Happenings programs allow hospital staff to support patients and help them understand what is going on medically. This information eases patients' fears and helps prepare them for the often difficult road ahead.

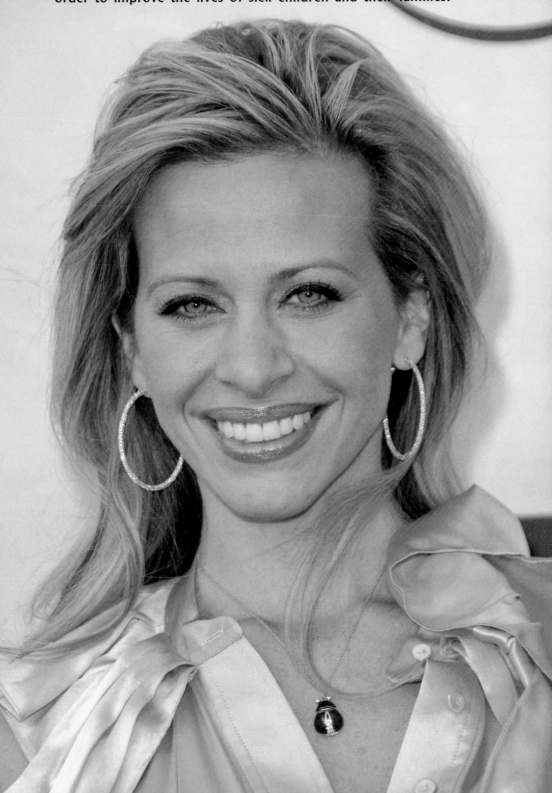

Television personality Dina Manzo started Project Ladybug in order to improve the lives of sick children and their families.

There are many creative ways to raise money for charity. The Smitheman family of Montreal, Canada, created a Haunted Yard during Halloween 2013 in order to raise money and awareness for the Starlight Foundation.

Today, the Starlight Foundation partners with more than 1,750 healthcare facilities and major pediatric hospitals around the world and serves millions of children every year.[3] Granting a wish, donating a card, or sending a letter can do more than just cheer up a patient for a few hours or a day. It can give that child and his or her family a ray of hope and a belief that good things can happen. It can also give a child the courage or motivation to keep fighting and endure the difficult treatments designed to make him or her well again.

As the founders of Project Ladybug, a charity that donates toys and arranges events to lift the spirits of children suffering from life-threatening illnesses, have said, "Our mission is clear. Through improving quality of life for these children and their families during treatment, PLB hopes to improve outcomes for these patients."[4]

A Gallery of Wishes

Here are just a few of the many wishes the Make-a-Wish Foundation granted in 2013:

- A little boy named Joe Joe got a set of cowboy gear, took part in a rodeo, and was named "Cowboy of the Year."

- Nicholas traveled to meet his favorite football team, the Minnesota Vikings, and had a Vikings-themed party.

- Nick appeared on the television show *Today*, where he was surprised by a visit from his hero, wrestler John Cena, who let him wear his championship belt.

- Janelle was an honorary manager of the Oakland A's for a day. Her duties included delivering the team's lineup for a game, meeting players, and touring the stadium.

- Aspiring baker Alexis was treated to a limo ride to a local bakery, where professional chefs taught her how to make cookies and other desserts.

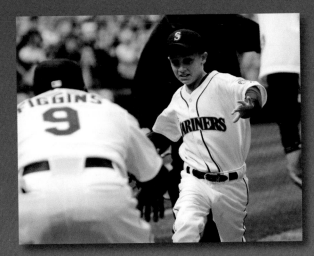

- Teenage basketball fan Thiago attended one of the Miami Heat's practices, worked out with the team, and had a basketball-shooting contest with superstar LeBron James.

Seattle Mariner Chone Figgins encourages nine-year-old kidney-transplant survivor Kyle Wolden to slide into home plate during a Make-a-Wish event before a Major League Baseball game in 2010.

- Sapphire had a Disney dream come true when she and her family traveled to Disney World and got to meet the Disney princesses.[5]

CHAPTER 5

Corporate Giving

It takes a lot of money to help sick children, and it takes a lot of people to help too. Many individuals volunteer their time and their money to organizations around the world, but there is always a need for more support, more workers, and more money. Fortunately, many major corporations have stepped up to help sick children.

The VoluntEARS

Disney movies and theme parks have made millions of children happy. However, the Walt Disney Company has another way to touch children's lives.

Disney encourages its employees to volunteer. These employees are called "VoluntEARS," after Mickey Mouse's famous ears. Disney estimates that since the program was founded, VoluntEARS have given nearly six million hours of service around the world.

Many times, VoluntEARS go into hospitals to donate Disney-themed books, games, and toys. Employees often go in costume as Disney characters. As Disney employee David Gill explains on the company's website, "I didn't know what to expect the first time I visited a hospital as a Disney VoluntEAR. Mickey, Minnie, and I walked in the door with toys in hand. The smiles we witnessed were priceless. I could see that the young patients were able to forget their worries—even if just for a moment—and be kids again."[1]

According to the Disney Company's website, Disney works to be a "positive and productive member of the community" by

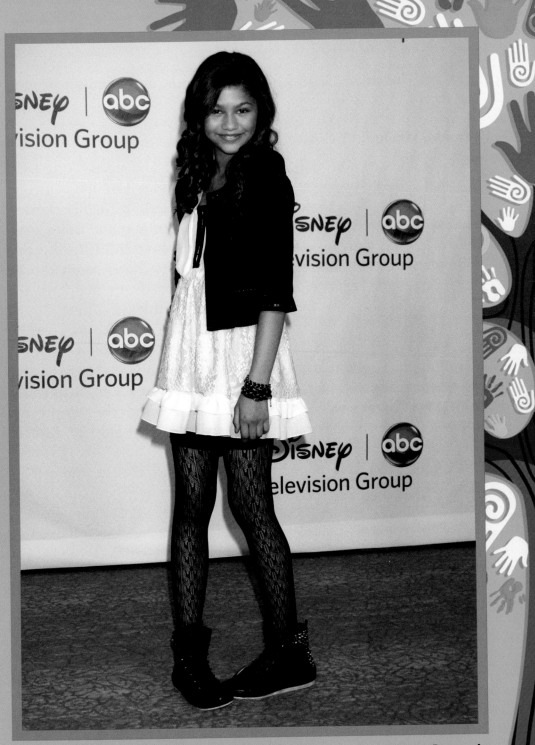

Disney star Zendaya Coleman at the ABC Summer Press Tour Party. In 2012, she joined Disney's VoluntEARS to give backpacks filled with school supplies to children in San Pedro, California.

bringing "positive, lasting change to kids and families around the world."[2]

Ronald McDonald House Charities

When a child is seriously ill or badly hurt and needs long-term hospital care, he or she is not the only person whose life is turned upside-down. The child's family also faces difficult choices, especially if the child has to travel to a hospital many miles from home. Parents naturally want to be with their child during this difficult time, but renting an apartment or a hotel room can be very expensive, especially if the family needs to maintain the family home and care for other children at the same time.

In 1974, McDonald's came up with an idea to help by creating the first Ronald McDonald House.[3] A Ronald McDonald House is a special place where families can live while their children receive treatment in hospitals. Ronald McDonald House Charities states that more than seven million families around the world are assisted by this charity every year while they stay in Ronald McDonald Houses in 58 countries.[4]

Families can stay at a Ronald McDonald House while their children are in the hospital and pay only what they can afford, even if that means paying nothing. Ronald McDonald Houses feature private rooms, kid-friendly playrooms, and staff that cares for families and even prepares hot, home-cooked meals for residents. Some Ronald McDonald Houses even arrange for educational services so children can stay up-to-date with their schoolwork while they are away from home, and also provide counseling and support services for siblings and other family members. Costs are taken care of through corporate giving and donations, including donation boxes set up in McDonald's restaurants.

Countless families have been helped by the comfort and support they found at Ronald McDonald Houses. Tripp Halstead's family spent six months at a Ronald McDonald House near Atlanta, Georgia, after the two-year-old was hit by a falling tree

Leukemia patient Mars Worsley shares a happy moment with his mother at a Ronald McDonald House. Mars' medical treatments meant he was unable to go home for Christmas in 2013, but his family was able to be together for the holiday thanks to the Ronald McDonald House.

Yao Ming, a Houston Rockets all-star, poses for a picture with elementary school students in 2012. Ming became a global spokesman for the Ronald McDonald House in 2012. Ming and other athletes are just a few of the many people, famous or not, who give their time to help sick children.

branch and suffered a severe brain injury. "The Ronald McDonald House gave us unconditional love," Tripp's mother wrote in the RMHC blog. "Above all, the House and its staff and volunteers gave us light. Even if I was dragging myself 'home' from the hospital at two in the morning, the House was never dark. There was always a smiling face at the door and a place to call home. It was a beacon of hope."[5]

Some hospitals don't have Ronald McDonald Houses nearby, but they have Ronald McDonald Family Rooms. These rooms are located in the hospitals themselves and provide a place for families to rest while caring for their sick children. Each Family Room features a place to sleep, shower, read, do laundry, or just sit and relax while watching TV or surfing the Internet.

Recently, McDonald's came up with a mobile health-care center called Ronald McDonald Care Mobile. This service features fully equipped medical vans that travel into remote or poor communities to provide a variety of services: everything from basic checkups to dental care, vision and hearing screenings, vaccinations, and nutrition information.[6]

Filling a Need

The need for public health care in poor communities is real. Here are some startling facts:

- More than 51 million hours of school are lost every year because of a lack of dental care among American children.[7]

- Tooth decay is the most common chronic disease in the United States. Asthma is second.[8]

- In Poland, 20 percent of childhood cancers are not diagnosed until they are in an advanced state.[9]

- In Latvia, almost ten percent of children have serious vision problems that prevent them from doing well in school or make everyday activities a challenge.[10]

- Nearly ten million children die worldwide every year of preventable and treatable causes.[11]

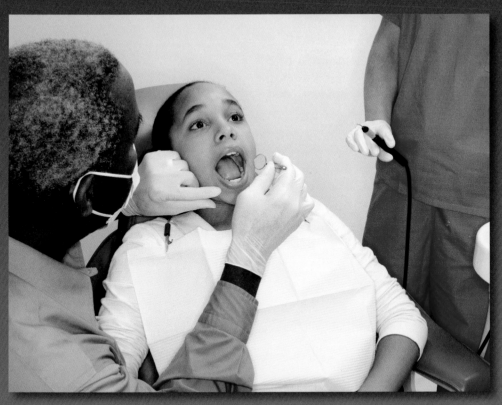

Child at dentist.

WHAT YOU CAN DO TO HELP

Childhood illnesses, injuries, and other hardships will never go away. However, by helping society's smallest members, millions of people have changed the world, one child at a time. We hope that after reading this book, you are inspired to help sick children. Here are some ideas:

Find a cause that is close to you. Perhaps you have a friend or relative who has a specific illness or disability and you've seen first-hand how difficult things can be for people with that condition. Helping is the most satisfying when you have a personal stake in the cause. Think about what matters to you and how you want to make a difference.

Start close to home. Ask your parents and teachers what local groups are in your area. For example, your police department may conduct a toy drive for hospitalized children, a local hospital might need volunteers to play with children being treated there, or a neighborhood group might be running a fundraiser such as a dinner or an auction to raise money for a child who needs medical treatment. You can also start your own fund-raising activities if you know someone who needs help (and have that person and their family's permission, of course). For example, a boy we know worked with the staff at his Catholic school to have students pay a small amount of money in exchange for an "out of uniform day." That money was donated to researching a cure for a disease that had claimed the life of the boy's best friend.

Do your research. If you want to support a larger cause, there is probably already a national organization that is working in the area. Check the books and databases at your local library to see who are the leaders in the field you're interested in, or do your own Internet research from home to find an organization you want to support.

Be creative! Short of donating your allowance or doing odd jobs to earn cash, how can you find money to donate to a cause you love? Think of creative ideas that you can do alone or with your friends. For example, you might ask a local store if you and your friends can do a collection drive outside the building. If you're artistic, perhaps you can make jewelry, artwork, or car magnets to sell and then donate your profits. Maybe you can write a blog or use social media to gain support. Check with your parents first to make sure your idea is safe and sensible, but don't be afraid to use your imagination!

Remember, you can donate more than money. Many organizations are looking for volunteers to work at fundraising events or just spread the word about a good cause. You can contact national and local organizations through their websites for more information. (Again, get your parents' permission first!)

Beware!

Many charities are dedicated to doing good work and helping others. However, there are other "charities" that aren't helping anyone but themselves. Fake charities are really scams that just want to take people's money and don't provide any assistance to sick children or organizations that help them. Other charities are poorly managed and although they mean well, they aren't set up to collect and donate money to the causes they're trying to help. It is always a good idea to research a charity or organization before getting involved with them. Here are some safe steps to take:

Do your research. Look at the charity's website and check other media outlets to see what they have to say about the charity or organization. There are many Websites that evaluate charities and report on how much money they actually give to the causes they support. Check out Charity Navigator (www.charitynavigator.org) or Charity Watch (www.charitywatch.org) to start with.

Talk to grownups. Before you commit your time or money or share your personal information with any organization, ask around. Check with your parents, teachers, and other adults you trust. What charities do they support?

Start locally. It's easier to know who to trust when your friends and neighbors are involved. There are many local organizations, from police departments to businesses to volunteer groups, at work in every community to make life better for sick children. Ask around and have the grownups in your life ask too. Be open to advice and be careful. Your time, money, and information are all very valuable, and the best way to help others is to use them wisely.

CHAPTER NOTES

Chapter 1: Batkid Makes a Wish

1. Ng, Christina. "Batkid's Make-a-Wish Transforms San Francisco Into Gotham." November 15, 2013. ABCNews.com. http://abcnews.go.com/US/batkids-make-transformed-san-francisco-gotham/story?id=20899254
2. Ibid.
3. Ibid.
4. Ibid.
5. Ibid.
6. Make-A-Wish America. http://wish.org

Chapter 2: Saving Young Lives Around the World

1. World Health Organization. http://www.who.int
2. Ibid.
3. Ibid.
4. UNICEF. http://unicef.org
5. Save the Children. http://www.savethechildren.net
6. Ibid.
7. Ibid.
8. EveryOne. http://everyone.savethechildren.net/about
9. Measles and Rubella Initiative. http://www.measlesrubellainitiative.org
10. Ibid.
11. Ibid.
12. Ibid.
13. Ibid.
14. Ibid.
15. Ibid.
16. Ibid.
17. Ibid.

Chapter 3: Medical Research and Care

1. St. Jude Children's Research Hospital. http://www.stjude.org
2. Ibid.
3. Shriners Hospitals for Children. http://www.shrinershospitalsforchildren.org

4. Ibid.
5. Ibid.
6. Ibid.
7. Ibid.
8. St. Jude Children's Research Hospital. http://www.stjude.org

Chapter 4: Fulfilling Wishes

1. Starlight Children's Foundation. http://www.starlight.org
2. Ibid.
3. Ibid.
4. Project Ladybug. http://www.projectladybug.org
5. Roth, Madeline. "17 Wishes The Make-a-Wish Foundation Has Granted This Year." July 22, 2013. Buzzfeed.com. http://www.buzzfeed.com/madroth/17-wishes-the-make-a-wish-foundation-has-granted-t-8tli

Chapter 5: Corporate Giving

1. Disney Post: The Official Blog of the Walt Disney Company. https://thewaltdisneycompany.com/blog/disney-delivers-care-packages-childrens-hospitals-around-world
2. Charitable Giving: The Walt Disney Company. http://thewaltdisneycompany.com/citizenship/community/charitable-giving
3. Ronald McDonald House Charities. http://www.rmhc.org
4. Ibid.
5. Ibid.
6. Ibid.
7. Ibid
8. Ibid.
9. Ibid.
10. Ibid.
11. Ibid.

FURTHER READING

Works Consulted

Charitable Giving: The Walt Disney Company http://thewaltdisneycompany.com/citizenship/community/charitable-giving

Disney Post: The Official Blog of the Walt Disney Company https://thewaltdisneycompany.com/blog/disney-delivers-care-packages-childrens-hospitals-around-world

FURTHER READING

EveryOne
http://everyone.savethechildren.net/about

Families of Children with Cancer: Volunteering at Children's Hospitals
http://www.fcco.org/helpvolunteer.html

Kids Helping Kids: Hope for Henry Foundation
http://www.hopeforhenry.org/kids-helping-kids

Make-A-Wish America
http://wish.org

Measles and Rubella Initiative
http://www.measlesrubellainitiative.org

Ng, Christina. "Batkid's Make-a-Wish Transforms San Francisco Into Gotham." November 15, 2013. ABCNews.com. http://abcnews.go.com/US/batkids-make-transformed-san-francisco-gotham/story?id=20899254

Project Ladybug
http://www.projectladybug.org

Ronald McDonald House Charities
http://www.rmhc.org

Roth, Madeline. "17 Wishes The Make-a-Wish Foundation Has Granted This Year." July 22, 2013. Buzzfeed.com. http://www.buzzfeed.com/madroth/17-wishes-the-make-a-wish-foundation-has-granted-t-8tli

Save the Children
http://www.savethechildren.net

Shriners Hospitals for Children
http://www.shrinershospitalsforchildren.org

Sparks, Rachelle. *Once Upon a Wish: True Inspirational Stories of Make-a-Wish Children.* Dallas, Texas: BenBella Books, Inc., 2013.

St. Jude Children's Research Hospital
http://www.stjude.org

Starlight Children's Foundation
http://www.starlight.org

UNICEF
http://www.unicef.org

World Health Organization
http://www.who.int

TIMELINE

1919   Save the Children is founded in London, England.

1922   The first Shriners Hospital for Children opens in Shreveport, Louisiana.

1946   UNICEF is formed.

1948   The World Health Organization is formed.

1958   The World Health Organization begins its campaign to eradicate smallpox.

1962   The first St. Jude Children's Research Hospital opens in Memphis, Tennessee; the Shriners open three hospitals to treat young burn patients.

1974   The first Ronald McDonald House opens.

1980   The Make-a-Wish Foundation is formed.

1981   The Make-a-Wish Foundation grants its first official wish.

1982   The Starlight Foundation is formed.

2000   The Measles and Rubella Initiative begins.

2015   The year the Every One campaign hopes to achieve a two-thirds reduction in child mortality.

2020   The year the Measles and Rubella Initiative hopes to eradicate measles.

GLOSSARY

catastrophic (kah-tass-TRAH-fik) — Something terrible.

clinical trials (KLIN-uh-kuhl TRY-uhls) — Medical treatments given to a group of patients to see how well the treatments work.

complications (kom-plih-KAY-shuhnz) — Events or issues that make things more difficult; another disease that develops as a result of the first illness.

contagious (kuhn-TAY-juhss) — A disease that is easy to catch.

corporate (KOR-puh-ruht) — Having to do with a business.

disabilities (diss-uh-BILL-uh-teez) — Restrictions on what a person can do caused by illness, injury, or birth defects.

donations (doh-NAY-shuhnz) — Money or gifts given to help someone.

eradicate (uh-RAD-uh-kate) — To wipe out completely.

foundation (foun-DAY-shuhn) — An organization that gives money to worthwhile causes.

fundraising (FUND-ray-zing) — Raising money for a cause or a charity.

grafting (GRAFT-ing) — Attaching living skin or tissue to replace damaged tissue.

immune (ih-MYOON) — Protected against a disease.

initiatives (ih-NISH-ee-uh-tivs) — Steps taken to achieve a result.

leukemia (loo-KEE-mee-uh) — A cancer that affects the blood.

mobile (MOH-buhl) — Able to move.

mortality (mor-TAL-uh-tee) — The number of deaths in a given time or place.

orthopedic (or-thuh-PEE-dik) — The branch of medicine having to do with bones and joints.

prosthetics (pros-THET-iks) — Artificial or mechanical limbs.

public health (PUB-lik HELTH) — Having to do with the health of an entire community.

rehabilitation (ree-hah-bill-ih-TAY-shuhn) — A program of exercises and therapy to help a person regain abilities after an injury or illness.

vaccination (vak-suh-NAY-shuhn) — An injection of medicine to help prevent disease.

volunteer (vol-uhn-TEER) — A person who does a job without pay.

INDEX

ABOUT THE AUTHOR

Joanne Mattern is the author of many books for children. She specializes in nonfiction and especially likes writing about people and animals. Joanne has written many books for Mitchell Lane, including biographies as well as several books about food and culture. She lives in New York State with her husband, children, and several pets.